METABOLICAL
MAELSTROM

Exposing the Deception in Processed Foods, Nutrition, and Medicine:

Unveiling the Hidden Truths Behind Our Food Choices and Health Misconceptions"

James K. Lamm

Disclaimer

Table Of Contents

Disclaimer..2

Introduction...7

The Seductive Allure of Processed Food...... 8

The Evolution of Modern Nutrition and
Medicine.. 11

Chapter 1..15

The Rise of Processed Food.......................... 15

Historical Context: From Farm to Factory.. 16

The Birth of Processed Food Industry Giants.
18

The Science of Food Processing.................20

Effects on Nutritional Quality.................... 22

Chapter 2..25

The Western Diet: A Recipe for Disaster...... 25

The Standard American Diet (SAD)........... 26

Health Implications of the Standard
American Diet... 28

Scientific Evidence and Case Studies..........31

Chapter 3..33

Unraveling the Nutritional Myth.................. 33

Nutrient Content vs. Nutrient Density.........34

Impact of Food Processing on Nutritional Composition....................................36

Deceptive Marketing Tactics....................39

Chapter 4...43

The Gut Microbiome: Nature's Inner Ecosystem..43

The Role of the Gut Microbiota in Overall Health...44

The Gut-Brain Axis, and Processed Food Consumption...46

How Processed Food Alters Gut Health......48

Chapter 5...51

Sugar: The Bitter Truth........................51

The Role of Sugar in the Diet.....................52

Hidden Sugars in Processed Foods.............54

The Addictive Nature of Sugar and Strategies for Reduction..55

Chapter 6...59

The Fat Fallacy.......................................59

Understanding Dietary Fats........................59

Saturated Fat, Cholesterol, and Heart Disease 64

The Low-Fat Myth.....................................68

Chapter 7...73

Beyond Calories: Hormones, Metabolism, and Weight Regulation...................................**73**

The Hormonal Impact of Processed Foods. 74

Insulin Resistance and Metabolic Syndrome.. 76

The Importance of Food Quality................. 78

Chapter 8...**81**

The Industrialization of Agriculture.............**81**

The Green Revolution and Its Consequences.. 82

Pesticides, Herbicides, and GMOs.............. 85

Sustainable Alternatives for Food Production. 88

Chapter 9...**91**

The Medicalization of Food......................... **91**

The Influence of Pharmaceutical Companies on Nutrition Research...................................92

Critique of Medications as a Band-Aid Solution for Dietary Diseases.....................94

Integrative Approaches to Health and Healing.. 97

Chapter 10..**101**

Navigating the Food Landscape:Practical Solutions for a Healthier Future................. **101**

   Strategies for Reducing Processed Food Consumption..102

   The Value of Whole Foods and Home Cooking... 106

   Advocacy for Policy Change and Food System Reform.. 111

Conclusion... **117**

Introduction

In the dimly lit aisles of a bustling supermarket, a seemingly endless array of colorful packages beckons shoppers with promises of convenience, flavor, and satisfaction. From crispy potato chips to sugary breakfast cereals, from microwave dinners to soda pop, processed foods dominate the shelves, filling carts and bellies alike. It's estimated that in the United States alone, approximately 70% of the average diet consists of processed foods. The allure of these products is undeniable they're quick, they're tasty, and they're everywhere. But as convenient as they may be, the consequences of our love affair with processed foods are becoming increasingly clear.

An Engaging Anecdote
Picture this: a family gathers around the dinner table, each member with a plate piled high with processed delicacies. The TV drones in the

background, forgotten in favor of the latest frozen pizza or fast-food creation. This scenario is all too familiar in modern households, where processed foods have become the cornerstone of daily meals. But what many fail to realize is that these seemingly harmless convenience foods often come with a hefty price tag and a toll on health that can be devastating if left unchecked.

The Seductive Allure of Processed Food

Processed food has become an integral part of modern life, offering convenience, affordability, and seemingly endless variety. From the brightly colored packaging lining supermarket shelves to the enticing aromas wafting from fast-food chains, processed foods exert a powerful allure that is hard to resist. But behind the glossy exterior lies a troubling reality: the seduction of processed food often comes at a significant cost to our health and well-being.

At its core, the appeal of processed food lies in its ability to tantalize our taste buds with a potent combination of salt, sugar, and fat. These three ingredients, known as the "holy trinity" of processed foods, are carefully calibrated to trigger pleasure centers in the brain, creating a sense of satisfaction and craving for more. Whether it's the crispy texture of a potato chip, the creamy sweetness of a chocolate bar, or the savory umami of a frozen pizza, processed foods are designed to be irresistible.

But the allure of processed food extends beyond its sensory appeal. In our fast-paced, hectic world, convenience is king and processed foods offer a quick and easy solution to the perennial question of what to eat. Busy schedules, long commutes, and demanding workloads leave little time or energy for meal preparation, making it all too tempting to reach for a pre-packaged meal or snack instead. And with advertising and marketing campaigns bombarding us at every turn, promoting the latest "must-have" food products, it's easy to succumb to the siren call of processed foods without fully considering their impact on our health.

Yet, as we indulge in the pleasures of processed food, we often overlook the hidden costs lurking beneath the surface. Processed foods are typically high in calories, refined carbohydrates, unhealthy fats, and sodium while lacking essential nutrients like fiber, vitamins, and minerals. Regular consumption of these nutrient-poor foods has been linked to a host of health problems, including obesity, diabetes, heart disease, and even certain types of cancer. What's more, the long-term health consequences of a diet high in processed foods can extend far beyond physical ailments, contributing to mental health issues such as depression, anxiety, and cognitive decline.

In today's hyper-connected world, the allure of processed food is stronger than ever, fueled by social media influencers, celebrity endorsements, and viral marketing campaigns.

But as we navigate the complex landscape of modern food choices, it's essential to pause and consider the true cost of our dietary decisions. By understanding the seductive allure of processed food and its impact on our health, we can empower ourselves to make informed choices that prioritize nourishment, vitality, and well-being.

The Evolution of Modern Nutrition and Medicine

The story of modern nutrition and medicine is one of remarkable progress and profound transformation. Over the past century, advances in science, technology, and medicine have revolutionized our understanding of human health and disease, paving the way for groundbreaking discoveries and life-saving interventions. Yet, alongside these triumphs, a darker narrative has emerged, characterized by the influence of vested interests, ideological agendas, and the relentless pursuit of profit at the expense of public health.

The roots of modern nutrition and medicine can be traced back to the early 20th century, a time of great optimism and innovation in the field of health and wellness. The discovery of essential vitamins and minerals laid the foundation for our understanding of nutrition, while the development of antibiotics and vaccines heralded a new era in the treatment and prevention of infectious diseases. These breakthroughs represented triumphs of human ingenuity and cooperation, offering hope for a future free from the scourge of illness and suffering.

Yet, as the 20th century progressed, the landscape of nutrition and medicine began to shift in profound and unexpected ways. The rise of industrialization and urbanization brought about profound changes in our diets and lifestyles, as traditional foodways gave way to the mass production and consumption of processed foods. Meanwhile, the pharmaceutical industry emerged as a powerful force in shaping medical practice and policy, wielding influence over everything from drug development to clinical guidelines to public health initiatives.

In this brave new world of modern nutrition and medicine, the lines between science, industry, and politics have become increasingly blurred, giving rise to conflicts of interest and ethical dilemmas that continue to plague the field today. From the promotion of fad diets and miracle cures to the suppression of inconvenient truths and dissenting voices, the pursuit of profit has often taken precedence over the pursuit of truth and public health.

Yet, Despite these hurdles, there is reason to hope. As awareness grows of the link between diet, lifestyle, and chronic disease, a growing movement is emerging to reclaim the narrative of health and wellness from the forces of commercialism and commodification. From grassroots organizations advocating for food system reform to healthcare practitioners championing a more holistic approach to healing, there is a growing realization that true health cannot be purchased or sold, but rather nourished from inside.

In the pages that follow, we will explore the complex interplay between processed food, nutrition, and modern medicine, shining a light on the lure and the lies that have shaped our understanding of health and wellness. By delving deep into the science, politics, and economics of food and medicine, we hope to empower you to make informed choices that promote health, vitality, and resilience in an increasingly uncertain world.

Chapter 1

The Rise of Processed Food

Processed food has become an integral part of the modern diet, shaping our eating habits, health outcomes, and even cultural norms. To understand its prevalence today, we must delve into its historical roots, exploring how it emerged as a dominant force in the food industry and its subsequent impact on society.

Historical Context: From Farm to Factory

The journey from farm to table has undergone a remarkable transformation over the past century. In the not-so-distant past, food was primarily sourced from local farms and markets, with communities relying on seasonal harvests and traditional preservation methods to sustain themselves. However, the advent of industrialization in the late 19th and early 20th centuries brought about profound changes in the way food was produced, processed, and distributed.

One of the key catalysts for this shift was the rise of urbanization, as people migrated from rural areas to cities in search of employment opportunities. As populations became increasingly concentrated in urban centers, the demand for food that could be mass-produced and transported over long distances grew exponentially. This demand, coupled with advancements in transportation and refrigeration technologies, paved the way for the industrialization of food production.

The Industrial Revolution ushered in an era of unprecedented innovation in agriculture and food processing. Traditional farming practices gave way to large-scale mechanized farming operations, where crops were grown monoculturally and chemical inputs such as fertilizers and pesticides became commonplace. These changes not only increased the efficiency of food production but also led to a significant expansion of the food supply.

Simultaneously, the emergence of food processing as an industry transformed the way food was prepared and packaged. In the early 20th century, pioneers like Clarence Birdseye and George A. Hormel revolutionized the food industry with inventions such as frozen food and canned meat products, respectively. These innovations not only extended the shelf life of perishable foods but also made them more accessible to consumers year-round.

The Birth of Processed Food Industry Giants

The consolidation of the food industry into a handful of multinational corporations is a phenomenon that has occurred relatively recently in human history. Over the past few decades, a small number of companies have come to dominate the global food market, wielding immense influence over what we eat and how our food is produced.

One of the most notable examples of this consolidation is the rise of companies like Nestlé, PepsiCo, and Kraft Heinz, which have built vast empires through mergers, acquisitions, and aggressive marketing tactics. These conglomerates control a significant portion of the world's food supply, producing everything from packaged snacks and beverages to frozen meals and condiments.

The consolidation of power within the food industry has raised concerns about market concentration and monopolistic practices. Critics argue that the dominance of a few major players stifles competition, limits consumer choice, and drives up prices. Moreover, the immense lobbying power of these corporations has enabled them to influence government policies and regulations in their favor, often at the expense of public health and environmental sustainability.

At the same time, the rise of processed food industry giants has been accompanied by a proliferation of highly processed, nutrient-poor foods. These products, which are often laden with artificial additives, preservatives, and flavor enhancers, have been linked to a host of health problems, including obesity, diabetes, and heart disease. Despite growing awareness of the health risks associated with processed foods, their convenience and affordability continue to make them a staple of modern diets.

The Science of Food Processing

At the heart of the processed food industry lies a sophisticated arsenal of food processing techniques designed to enhance flavor, texture, and shelf life while maximizing profitability. From extrusion and emulsification to dehydration and fermentation, these methods transform raw ingredients into a dizzying array of packaged products that populate grocery store aisles.

Extrusion, for example, is a ubiquitous process used to produce breakfast cereals, snack foods, and pet kibble. This high-pressure, high-temperature method involves forcing a mixture of grains, starches, and additives through a die to create uniform shapes and textures. While extrusion offers unparalleled efficiency and consistency, critics argue that the process can denature proteins, degrade vitamins, and produce harmful compounds like acrylamide.

Emulsification, on the other hand, is a technique used to create stable suspensions of oil and water, giving rise to creamy salad dressings, smooth mayonnaise, and velvety ice cream. By combining hydrophilic and hydrophobic molecules through mechanical agitation or chemical emulsifiers, manufacturers can achieve the desired texture and mouthfeel, even in low-fat or fat-free formulations.

Dehydration, a time-honored method of food preservation, involves removing moisture from foods through evaporation or freeze-drying, extending their shelf life and portability. From dried fruits and jerky to instant noodles and powdered soup mixes, dehydrated products offer convenience without sacrificing flavor or nutrition.

Fermentation, perhaps one of the oldest forms of food processing, harnesses the power of microorganisms to transform raw ingredients into flavorful and nutritious delicacies. Yogurt, cheese, sauerkraut, and sourdough bread are just a few examples of fermented foods that have graced tables around the world for centuries, providing essential nutrients, beneficial bacteria, and unique culinary experiences.

Effects on Nutritional Quality

While food processing has undoubtedly revolutionized the way we eat, its impact on the nutritional quality of our diet remains a subject of debate and scrutiny. On one hand, processing can enhance the bioavailability of certain nutrients, improve food safety, and extend the shelf life of perishable goods, thereby reducing food waste and increasing access to affordable nutrition.

On the other hand, many processing techniques strip foods of their natural vitamins, minerals, and fiber, while adding excessive amounts of salt, sugar, and artificial additives. The proliferation of ultra-processed foods, characterized by long ingredient lists and minimal whole ingredients, has been linked to a host of diet-related health problems, including obesity, diabetes, heart disease, and cancer.

Moreover, the relentless pursuit of profit and market share has led some manufacturers to prioritize taste, texture, and shelf stability over nutritional integrity, resulting in a flood of hyper-palatable, nutrient-poor products that contribute to the global burden of malnutrition and chronic disease. As consumers become increasingly aware of the link between diet and health, there is a growing demand for minimally processed, whole foods that nourish the body and support overall well-being.

Chapter 2

The Western Diet:

A Recipe for Disaster

The Standard American Diet (SAD) has become emblematic of modern eating habits in the Western world. Characterized by high levels of processed foods, refined sugars, unhealthy fats, and low intake of fruits, vegetables, and whole grains, the SAD represents a significant departure from traditional diets that prioritized fresh, whole foods. In this chapter, we will explore the defining characteristics of the SAD and its profound implications for public health. Through the lens of scientific evidence and real-life case studies, we will illuminate the direct link between processed food consumption and the alarming rise in obesity, diabetes, and cardiovascular disease.

The Standard American Diet (SAD)

At the core of the SAD lies a reliance on highly processed, nutrient-poor foods that are engineered for taste, convenience, and shelf-life rather than nutritional value. These foods are typically high in refined carbohydrates, added sugars, unhealthy fats, and sodium, while lacking in essential vitamins, minerals, and dietary fiber. Let's delve into some of the key characteristics of the SAD:

1. **High Consumption of Processed Foods**: Processed foods, including ready-to-eat meals, snacks, sugary beverages, and fast food items, constitute a significant portion of the SAD. These foods are often laden with artificial

additives, preservatives, and flavor enhancers to prolong shelf life and enhance palatability.

2. **Excessive Sugar Intake**: Sugar is ubiquitous in the SAD, hidden in a myriad of processed foods under various names such as sucrose, high fructose corn syrup, and dextrose. From sugary breakfast cereals to soft drinks to baked goods, many staple items in the modern diet contribute to excessive sugar consumption, far exceeding recommended limits.

3. **Low Fruit and Vegetable Consumption**: Despite the well-documented health benefits of fruits and vegetables, the average American falls short of meeting daily recommendations. The SAD tends to prioritize processed foods over fresh produce, leading to inadequate intake of essential vitamins, minerals, and antioxidants crucial for overall health.

4. **High Intake of Unhealthy Fats**: The SAD is characterized by an overabundance of unhealthy fats, particularly trans fats and saturated fats,

derived from fried foods, processed meats, and commercially baked goods. These fats not only contribute to weight gain but also increase the risk of cardiovascular disease and other chronic conditions.

5. **Overreliance on Convenience Foods**: Busy lifestyles and the ubiquity of fast-food chains have normalized the consumption of convenience foods high in calories, sodium, and unhealthy additives. These convenient options often displace home-cooked meals made from scratch with wholesome ingredients.

Health Implications of the Standard American Diet

The consequences of the SAD extend far beyond mere dietary choices, exerting a profound impact on public health and well-being. Scientific research has unequivocally linked the consumption of processed foods typical of SAD to a host of chronic diseases, including obesity, diabetes, and cardiovascular disease. Let's examine each of these health implications in detail:

1. Obesity: The SAD's emphasis on calorie-dense, nutrient-poor foods contributes to excessive calorie intake and weight gain. Processed foods, high in refined sugars and unhealthy fats, promote overeating by disrupting hormonal signals that regulate appetite and satiety. Consequently, obesity rates have surged in recent decades, with more than two-thirds of American adults classified as overweight or obese.

2. Diabetes: The rapid rise in obesity rates driven by the SAD has paralleled a surge in type 2 diabetes cases. Diets rich in processed foods and added sugars promote insulin resistance, a hallmark of type 2 diabetes, wherein cells become less responsive to insulin signals, leading to elevated blood sugar levels. As a result, millions of individuals grapple with the debilitating consequences of uncontrolled diabetes, including cardiovascular complications, nerve damage, and kidney failure.

3. Cardiovascular Disease: The SAD's high sodium, saturated fat, and trans fat content exact a toll on cardiovascular health, contributing to the development of hypertension, atherosclerosis, heart attacks, and strokes. Processed foods laden with sodium, preservatives, and artificial additives not only raise blood pressure but also promote inflammation and oxidative stress, driving the progression of cardiovascular disease.

Scientific Evidence and Case Studies

The link between the Standard American Diet and its adverse health outcomes is substantiated by a wealth of scientific research spanning decades. Numerous epidemiological studies, clinical trials, and meta-analyses have consistently demonstrated the deleterious effects of processed food consumption on obesity, diabetes, and cardiovascular health.

For instance, a landmark study published in the Journal of the American Medical Association (JAMA) analyzed dietary patterns and health outcomes among a cohort of over 200,000 participants. The researchers found that adherence to a Western dietary pattern characterized by high intake of processed foods, red meat, and sugary beverages was associated with a significantly elevated risk of obesity, type 2 diabetes, and coronary artery disease.

Moreover, real-life case studies underscore the devastating toll of the SAD on individual health and quality of life. Consider the story of Sarah, a 45-year-old woman grappling with obesity, prediabetes, and hypertension. Despite numerous attempts to lose weight through fad diets and exercise regimens, Sarah's reliance on processed convenience foods continued to thwart her efforts, exacerbating her metabolic dysfunction and increasing her risk of chronic disease.

Similarly, the documentary Fed Up sheds light on the pervasive influence of the food industry on dietary habits and public health. Through compelling narratives and expert interviews, the film exposes the role of processed foods and sugary beverages in fueling the obesity epidemic and highlights the urgent need for systemic changes to address the root causes of poor dietary habits.

The Standard American Diet represents a recipe for disaster, fueling an epidemic of obesity, diabetes, and cardiovascular disease.

Chapter 3

Unraveling the Nutritional Myth

Nutrition is a cornerstone of human health, influencing every aspect of our well-being from physical vitality to mental acuity. Yet, in our modern era dominated by convenience and processed foods, the true essence of nutrition has become obscured by misleading labels, deceptive marketing tactics, and a general misunderstanding of what constitutes a truly nourishing diet. In this chapter, we delve into the heart of the nutritional myth, shedding light on the crucial differences between nutrient content and nutrient density, exploring how food processing alters the nutritional composition of foods, and exposing the deceptive marketing practices employed by the processed food industry.

Nutrient Content vs. Nutrient Density

Nutrient content and nutrient density are terms often used interchangeably, yet they represent distinct concepts that are fundamental to understanding the nutritional value of foods. Nutrient content simply refers to the amount of specific nutrients present in a given food item. This can be measured in terms of macronutrients such as carbohydrates, proteins, and fats, as well as micronutrients like vitamins and minerals.

On the other hand, nutrient density takes into account not only the quantity of nutrients in a food but also the quality and bioavailability of those nutrients relative to the total energy (caloric) content of the food. In other words, nutrient-dense foods provide a high concentration of essential nutrients per calorie, whereas nutrient-poor foods may contain a significant amount of calories but offer little in the way of essential vitamins, minerals, and other vital nutrients.

For example, a candy bar and a piece of fruit may contain a similar number of calories, but the fruit is considered more nutrient-dense because it provides a wealth of vitamins, minerals, fiber, and phytonutrients that support optimal health and vitality. In contrast, the candy bar is loaded with empty calories from refined sugars and unhealthy fats, offering little in the way of nutritional benefit.

Understanding the distinction between nutrient content and nutrient density is crucial for making informed dietary choices that promote health and longevity. By prioritizing nutrient-dense foods such as fruits, vegetables, whole grains, lean proteins, and healthy fats, individuals can ensure that they are meeting their nutritional needs while minimizing their intake of empty calories and processed junk foods.

Impact of Food Processing on Nutritional Composition

Food processing is a ubiquitous aspect of modern food production, encompassing a wide range of techniques designed to extend shelf life, enhance flavor and texture, and increase convenience. While some processing methods may have minimal impact on the nutritional quality of foods, others can significantly alter their nutrient composition, leading to a reduction in overall nutrient density.

One of the most common ways in which food processing affects nutritional quality is through the removal or destruction of essential nutrients during refining and manufacturing processes. For example, the milling of grains to produce white flour strips away the bran and germ layers, which are rich in fiber, vitamins, minerals, and phytonutrients. What remains is a refined carbohydrate devoid of most of its original nutritional value.

Similarly, processing methods such as high-heat cooking, frying, and deep-frying can degrade heat-sensitive vitamins and denature proteins, reducing the bioavailability of nutrients and diminishing their health-promoting effects. Additionally, the addition of artificial preservatives, flavorings, and colorings in processed foods may further compromise their nutritional integrity, contributing to a host of health problems ranging from nutrient deficiencies to chronic diseases.

In recent years, there has been a growing awareness of the negative health consequences associated with excessive consumption of ultra-processed foods, which are typically high in sugar, unhealthy fats, sodium, and chemical additives. These highly palatable, calorie-dense foods not only displace more nutrient-dense options from the diet but also promote overeating and weight gain, leading to a cascade of metabolic disturbances and chronic health conditions.

As consumers become increasingly savvy about the detrimental effects of food processing on nutritional quality, there has been a resurgence of interest in whole, minimally processed foods that retain their natural goodness and nutritional integrity. By embracing a diet rich in fruits, vegetables, whole grains, legumes, nuts, seeds, and lean proteins, individuals can nourish their bodies with the essential nutrients they need to thrive while minimizing their exposure to harmful additives and empty calories.

Deceptive Marketing Tactics

In the competitive landscape of the food industry, marketing plays a pivotal role in shaping consumer perceptions and driving purchasing decisions. Unfortunately, many processed food companies have employed deceptive marketing tactics to promote their products as healthy or nutritious, despite evidence to the contrary. From misleading packaging claims to manipulative advertising campaigns, these tactics serve to obfuscate the truth about the nutritional quality of processed foods and perpetuate the myth that convenience equals health.

One common strategy used by the processed food industry is the use of health claims and buzzwords to create the illusion of nutritional superiority. Terms like "all-natural," "low-fat," "gluten-free," and "fortified with vitamins and minerals" are often plastered across packaging to convey a sense of wholesomeness and wellness. However, closer inspection reveals that many of these products are loaded with sugar, unhealthy fats, sodium, and artificial additives, which can have detrimental effects on health when consumed in excess.

Furthermore, the use of misleading imagery and language in advertising can further reinforce the perception that processed foods are a quick and easy solution to dietary woes. By associating their products with images of happy, healthy families and idyllic outdoor settings, food companies create an emotional connection with consumers and position their products as indispensable staples of modern living.

Another deceptive marketing tactic employed by the processed food industry is the manipulation of portion sizes and serving suggestions to downplay the true caloric and nutritional content of their products. By presenting unrealistic serving sizes and obscuring the total calorie count per package, companies can give the impression that their products are lower in calories and healthier than they actually are.

In recent years, regulatory agencies and consumer advocacy groups have taken steps to curb deceptive marketing practices in the food industry, but there is still much work to be done to ensure that consumers are not misled by false or exaggerated claims. By educating themselves about how to read food labels, decipher marketing jargon, and discern fact from fiction, individuals can make more informed choices about the foods they purchase and consume.

Unraveling the nutritional myth requires a critical examination of the differences between nutrient content and nutrient density, an understanding of how food processing alters the nutritional composition of foods, and a recognition of the deceptive marketing tactics employed by the processed food industry. By prioritizing whole, minimally processed foods and becoming savvy consumers, individuals can reclaim their health and well-being in an age of nutritional confusion and misinformation.

Chapter 4

The Gut Microbiome: Nature's Inner Ecosystem

The human body is a complex ecosystem teeming with trillions of microorganisms, collectively known as the microbiota, that inhabit various parts of our anatomy. Among these, the gut microbiota, residing primarily in the gastrointestinal tract, plays a pivotal role in maintaining our overall health and well-being. Comprising a diverse array of bacteria, fungi, viruses, and other microbes, the gut microbiome forms a dynamic ecosystem that interacts intricately with our body's physiology and immune system.

The Role of the Gut Microbiota in Overall Health

The gut microbiota is often referred to as our "second brain" due to its profound influence on various aspects of our health, ranging from digestion and nutrient absorption to immune function and mental well-being. This complex microbial community performs a multitude of essential functions, such as breaking down dietary fibers, synthesizing vitamins, metabolizing drugs, and protecting against pathogens.

One of the key functions of the gut microbiome is its involvement in the fermentation of dietary fibers and other indigestible carbohydrates. Through this process, beneficial bacteria in the gut produce short-chain fatty acids (SCFAs), such as butyrate, acetate, and propionate, which serve as an energy source for the cells lining the intestinal wall. SCFAs also exert anti-inflammatory effects and help maintain the integrity of the gut barrier, thereby preventing the leakage of harmful substances into the bloodstream.

Furthermore, the gut microbiota plays a crucial role in educating and regulating the immune system. By interacting with immune cells in the gut-associated lymphoid tissue (GALT), microbial communities help distinguish between harmless antigens and potentially harmful pathogens, thus preventing inappropriate immune responses and autoimmune reactions.

Moreover, emerging research has uncovered a fascinating link between the gut microbiome and mental health, highlighting the bidirectional communication between the gut and the brain known as the gut-brain axis. This communication occurs via various pathways, including the vagus nerve, neurotransmitters, and microbial metabolites, and has profound implications for mood, cognition, and behavior.

The Gut-Brain Axis, and Processed Food Consumption

The intricate interplay between gut health, the gut-brain axis, and dietary habits has garnered increasing attention from researchers and healthcare professionals alike. Of particular interest is the impact of processed food consumption on the composition and function of the gut microbiome, and its subsequent implications for both physical and mental health.

Processed foods, characterized by their high levels of refined sugars, unhealthy fats, artificial additives, and preservatives, represent a significant departure from the nutrient-dense, whole foods that our ancestors consumed for millennia. While these convenient and palatable products may satisfy our taste buds and satiate our hunger temporarily, they often take a toll on our gut health and microbial diversity in the long run.

Numerous studies have demonstrated that diets rich in processed foods can lead to dysbiosis, an imbalance in the gut microbiota characterized by a reduction in beneficial bacteria and an overgrowth of potentially harmful microbes. This dysbiotic state is associated with various gastrointestinal disorders, including irritable bowel syndrome (IBS), inflammatory bowel disease (IBD), and leaky gut syndrome, as well as systemic conditions such as obesity, type 2 diabetes, and cardiovascular disease.

Furthermore, the consumption of processed foods has been shown to disrupt the delicate equilibrium of the gut-brain axis, potentially contributing to mood disorders such as depression and anxiety. Research suggests that alterations in gut microbial composition and metabolite production can influence neurotransmitter signaling, neuroinflammation, and stress response pathways, thereby affecting mood and cognitive function.

How Processed Food Alters Gut Health

The detrimental effects of processed foods on gut microbiome composition and function are multifaceted and encompass several mechanisms. Firstly, these ultra-processed products are often devoid of dietary fibers, prebiotics, and other nutrients that support the growth and diversity of beneficial bacteria in the gut. Instead, they are laden with refined sugars, which serve as a substrate for pathogenic microbes and promote dysbiosis.

Additionally, many processed foods contain artificial additives, emulsifiers, and preservatives that can disrupt the gut barrier function and trigger inflammatory responses in susceptible individuals. These additives may alter the mucus layer lining the intestinal epithelium, compromise tight junction integrity, and promote the translocation of bacteria and toxins across the gut barrier, leading to systemic inflammation and metabolic dysfunction.

Moreover, the high fat and calorie content of processed foods can contribute to obesity and metabolic syndrome, conditions that are closely linked to alterations in gut microbiome composition and function. Excessive consumption of saturated fats and hydrogenated oils found in processed snacks, fast food, and packaged meals can promote the growth of pro-inflammatory bacteria while suppressing beneficial species, thereby perpetuating a cycle of dysbiosis and metabolic dysregulation.

The gut microbiome represents a complex and dynamic ecosystem that plays a crucial role in maintaining our overall health and well-being. However, the modern diet, characterized by the widespread consumption of processed foods, poses significant challenges to gut health and microbial diversity. By understanding the connection between gut health, the gut-brain axis, and dietary habits, we can take proactive steps to support our microbiome and promote optimal health through mindful food choices and lifestyle modifications.

Chapter 5

Sugar: The Bitter Truth

Sugar: The Sweet Saboteur

Sugar, once hailed as the epitome of sweetness, has now emerged as one of the most insidious components of the modern diet. Its prevalence in processed foods, combined with its addictive properties, has led to a cascade of health issues, ranging from obesity to diabetes and cardiovascular disease. In this chapter, we delve into the multifaceted role of sugar in the diet, uncover the hidden sugars lurking in processed foods, and explore strategies for curbing sugar consumption to reclaim our metabolic health.

The Role of Sugar in the Diet

Sugar, in its various forms such as sucrose, fructose, and glucose, is a ubiquitous ingredient in the modern food supply. While naturally occurring sugars in fruits and vegetables can be part of a healthy diet when consumed in moderation, the excessive consumption of added sugars, particularly in processed foods, poses significant health risks.

One of the primary functions of sugar in the diet is to provide a quick source of energy for the body. When consumed, sugars are rapidly absorbed into the bloodstream, causing a spike in blood glucose levels. In response, the pancreas releases insulin to facilitate the uptake of glucose into cells for energy production. However, frequent consumption of high-sugar foods can lead to insulin resistance, where cells become less responsive to insulin signals, ultimately contributing to the development of type 2 diabetes.

Moreover, sugar consumption has been linked to weight gain and obesity. Unlike whole foods that contain fiber, protein, and fats, which promote satiety and regulate appetite, sugary foods are often low in nutrients and fail to provide long-lasting feelings of fullness. As a result, individuals may consume excess calories from sugary snacks and beverages, leading to weight gain over time.

Furthermore, sugar has been implicated in various metabolic disturbances, including dyslipidemia, non-alcoholic fatty liver disease (NAFLD), and cardiovascular disease. Excessive sugar intake can elevate triglyceride levels, promote the accumulation of fat in the liver, and contribute to inflammation and oxidative stress, all of which are risk factors for heart disease.

Hidden Sugars in Processed Foods

Despite growing awareness of the health risks associated with sugar consumption, many individuals are unaware of the hidden sugars lurking in processed foods. Manufacturers often use a variety of sweeteners, such as high-fructose corn syrup, dextrose, and maltose, to enhance the flavor of packaged foods and beverages.

Common culprits include sugary breakfast cereals, flavored yogurt, granola bars, canned soups, and condiments like ketchup and barbecue sauce. Even seemingly healthy options, such as fruit-flavored yogurt and sports drinks, can contain staggering amounts of added sugars.

The pervasive presence of hidden sugars in processed foods not only contributes to excess calorie intake but also undermines efforts to maintain a balanced diet. Consumers may unknowingly consume large quantities of sugar throughout the day, exceeding recommended intake levels and increasing their risk of metabolic health issues.

Furthermore, the marketing tactics employed by food manufacturers can be deceptive, portraying sugary products as wholesome and nutritious choices. Terms like "natural," "low-fat," and "organic" may create a false sense of healthfulness, diverting attention away from the high sugar content of these products.

The Addictive Nature of Sugar and Strategies for Reduction

Sugar's addictive properties have been compared to those of drugs like cocaine and nicotine, eliciting cravings and reinforcing compulsive consumption behaviors. The consumption of sugary foods triggers the release of dopamine, a neurotransmitter associated with pleasure and reward, in the brain's reward centers. Over time, repeated exposure to high levels of sugar can lead to desensitization of dopamine receptors, requiring progressively larger doses of sugar to achieve the same level of pleasure.

Breaking free from the grip of sugar addiction requires a multifaceted approach that addresses both the physiological and psychological aspects of cravings. Below are some strategies for reducing sugar consumption and regaining control over your health:

- **Read Labels**: Become a vigilant label reader and scrutinize the ingredients list for hidden sugars. Look out for terms like sucrose, high-fructose corn syrup, cane juice, and evaporated cane juice, among others.

- **Choose Whole Foods**: Opt for whole, minimally processed foods whenever possible. Fruits, vegetables, whole grains, legumes, nuts, and seeds are naturally low in added sugars and packed with essential nutrients.

- **Cook at Home**: Take charge of your meals by preparing homemade dishes using fresh ingredients. Cooking from scratch allows you to control the amount of sugar and other additives in your food, ensuring a healthier outcome.

- **Practice Mindful Eating**: Pay attention to your body's hunger and fullness cues, and eat with awareness rather than on autopilot. Mindful eating can help you differentiate between physical hunger and emotional cravings, reducing the likelihood of impulsive sugar consumption.

- **Gradually Reduce Intake**: Instead of attempting to eliminate sugar from your diet overnight, start by gradually reducing your intake. Set realistic goals and make small, sustainable changes over time to avoid feelings of deprivation and withdrawal.

- **Find Healthy Alternatives**: Experiment with natural sweeteners like stevia, monk fruit, and erythritol as alternatives to refined sugar. While these sweeteners should be used in moderation, they can satisfy your sweet tooth without causing the same metabolic disturbances as sugar.

By adopting these strategies and cultivating a mindful approach to eating, you can reduce your sugar intake, support your metabolic health, and pave the way for long-term well-being. Sugar's pervasive presence in the modern diet poses significant challenges to metabolic health and overall well-being. By raising awareness of the role of sugar in the diet, identifying hidden sources of sugar in processed foods, and implementing strategies for reducing sugar consumption, individuals can take proactive steps to reclaim control over their health and break free from the cycle of sugar addiction.

Chapter 6

The Fat Fallacy

Understanding Dietary Fats

Dietary fats have long been demonized in popular culture and media, often portrayed as the enemy of health and weight loss. However, the reality is far more nuanced. Fats are essential macronutrients that play crucial roles in our bodies, from providing energy to supporting cell structure and hormone production. Understanding the different types of dietary fats and their effects on health is essential for making informed dietary choices.

Types of Dietary Fats:

There are several types of dietary fats, each with unique chemical structures and physiological effects:

Saturated Fats: Saturated fats are typically solid at room temperature and are found in foods such as meat, dairy products, and tropical oils like coconut and palm oil. They have been vilified for decades, with conventional wisdom linking them to heart disease. However, recent research suggests that the relationship between saturated fat intake and heart health is more complex than previously thought.

Monounsaturated Fats: Monounsaturated fats are liquid at room temperature and are found in foods like olive oil, avocados, and nuts. They are known for their heart-healthy benefits, including improving cholesterol levels and reducing the risk of cardiovascular disease.

Polyunsaturated fats: Omega-3 and omega-6 fatty acids are examples of polyunsaturated fats, which are also liquid at room temperature. Sources of polyunsaturated fats include fatty fish, seeds, and vegetable oils. Omega-3 fatty acids, in particular, are associated with numerous health benefits, including reducing inflammation and supporting brain health.

Trans Fats: Trans fats are artificial fats created through the process of hydrogenation, which makes liquid vegetable oils solid at room temperature. Trans fats are found in many processed and fried foods and have been linked to an increased risk of heart disease and other health problems. In recent years, there has been a push to reduce or eliminate trans fats from the food supply.

The Role of Dietary Fats in Health

Despite their bad reputation, dietary fats are essential for overall health and well-being. They provide a concentrated source of energy, with each gram of fat containing nine calories, compared to just four calories per gram of carbohydrates or protein. In addition to providing energy, fats are necessary for the absorption of fat-soluble vitamins (A, D, E, and K) and for the synthesis of hormones and cell membranes.

The type of fat consumed can have a significant impact on health outcomes. While excessive intake of saturated and trans fats has been linked to an increased risk of heart disease and other chronic conditions, replacing these fats with healthier alternatives like monounsaturated and polyunsaturated fats can have positive effects on cardiovascular health.

Making Healthy Fat Choices

When it comes to dietary fats, quality is key. Instead of focusing solely on reducing total fat intake, it's important to prioritize the consumption of healthy fats while minimizing the intake of unhealthy fats. Some tips for making healthy fat choices include:

- **Choose Whole Foods**: Opt for whole food sources of fat, such as avocados, nuts, seeds, and fatty fish, rather than processed or fried foods high in unhealthy fats.

- **Use Healthy Cooking Oils**: Cook with oils that are high in monounsaturated or polyunsaturated fats, such as olive oil, avocado oil, or walnut oil, instead of oils high in saturated or trans fats.

- **Read Labels**: Check food labels for hidden sources of unhealthy fats, such as partially hydrogenated oils, and avoid products containing trans fats whenever possible.

- **Limit Saturated Fat Intake**: While saturated fats are not as harmful as once believed, it's still wise to limit intake from sources like red meat and full-fat dairy products and instead focus on incorporating more plant-based fats into your diet.

By making informed choices and prioritizing the consumption of healthy fats, you can support your overall health and reduce your risk of chronic disease.

Saturated Fat, Cholesterol, and Heart Disease

For decades, saturated fat has been singled out as a dietary villain, with public health campaigns urging people to reduce their intake to prevent heart disease. This fear was largely based on the hypothesis that saturated fat raises cholesterol levels, particularly LDL cholesterol, which is commonly referred to as "bad" cholesterol, and contributes to the development of atherosclerosis and coronary artery disease. However, recent research has challenged this hypothesis and raised questions about the role of saturated fat in heart health.

The Saturated Fat-Cholesterol Connection

Saturated fat has long been believed to raise levels of LDL cholesterol, which is associated with an increased risk of heart disease. However, more recent research suggests that the relationship between saturated fat intake, cholesterol levels, and heart disease risk is more complex than previously thought.

While it's true that saturated fat can raise LDL cholesterol levels, it also tends to raise levels of HDL cholesterol, often referred to as "good" cholesterol, which has protective effects on heart health. Additionally, the size and density of LDL particles may be more important than the total

LDL cholesterol level when it comes to assessing heart disease risk.

The Role of Cholesterol in Heart Disease

Cholesterol is a waxy substance found in the blood and is essential for various physiological functions, including the production of hormones and the maintenance of cell membranes. However, high levels of LDL cholesterol can lead to the buildup of plaque in the arteries, a condition known as atherosclerosis, which increases the risk of heart attack and stroke.

While dietary saturated fat can influence cholesterol levels to some extent, genetics, lifestyle factors, and overall dietary patterns also play significant roles. For example, a diet high in refined carbohydrates and sugars may have a more detrimental effect on heart health than a diet high in saturated fat.

Reevaluating Dietary Recommendations

In light of emerging evidence, some experts have called for a reevaluation of dietary recommendations regarding saturated fat intake. Rather than focusing solely on reducing saturated fat intake, they argue that it's more important to prioritize whole, nutrient-dense foods and to consider the overall dietary pattern, including the consumption of fruits, vegetables, whole grains, and lean proteins.

Instead of demonizing saturated fat, the emphasis should be on reducing the consumption of processed foods high in refined carbohydrates, sugars, and unhealthy fats, which are more strongly associated with heart disease risk.

Ultimately, individualized dietary recommendations based on factors such as genetics, cholesterol levels, and overall health status may be more appropriate than blanket recommendations to reduce saturated fat intake for everyone. More research is needed to better understand the complex relationship between dietary fats, cholesterol levels, and heart disease risk.

The Low-Fat Myth

The low-fat diet craze took the world by storm in the late 20th century, fueled by public health campaigns and food industry marketing efforts promoting low-fat and fat-free products as the key to weight loss and heart health. However, despite decades of dietary recommendations to reduce fat intake, rates of obesity and chronic disease continued to rise, leading many to question the effectiveness and validity of the low-fat paradigm.

The Origins of the Low-Fat Movement

The low-fat diet trend gained momentum in the 1970s and 1980s, spurred by influential government reports and public health initiatives aimed at reducing heart disease rates. The prevailing belief was that dietary fat, particularly saturated fat, was the primary dietary culprit behind heart disease and obesity, and that reducing fat intake would lead to improved health outcomes.

As a result, food manufacturers began producing a plethora of low-fat and fat-free products, often replacing fat with sugar, refined carbohydrates, and artificial additives to improve taste and texture.

The Pitfalls of Low-Fat Diets

While reducing saturated fat intake may have some benefits for heart health, the low-fat diet craze led to several unintended consequences:

- Increased Sugar Consumption: Many low-fat and fat-free products are high in added sugars and refined carbohydrates, which can contribute to weight gain, insulin resistance, and metabolic dysfunction.

- Nutrient Deficiencies: Fat plays a crucial role in the absorption of fat-soluble vitamins (A, D, E, and K), as well as other essential nutrients. A low-fat diet may increase the risk of nutrient deficiencies, particularly in vitamins and minerals that are found in fat-rich foods.

- Unsustainability: Low-fat diets are often difficult to maintain in the long term due to feelings of hunger and deprivation. Restricting fat intake may also lead to cravings and overeating, ultimately undermining weight loss efforts.

The Shift Towards a Balanced Approach

In recent years, there has been a shift away from the low-fat paradigm towards a more balanced approach to nutrition. Rather than demonizing all fats, the focus is now on choosing healthy fats and prioritizing whole, minimally processed foods.

Instead of fixating on fat grams, dietary recommendations now emphasize the importance of overall dietary patterns, including the consumption of fruits, vegetables, whole grains, lean proteins, and healthy fats. The Mediterranean diet, for example, which is rich in monounsaturated fats from olive oil, nuts, and seeds, has been shown to reduce the risk of heart disease and other chronic conditions.

By adopting a more balanced approach to nutrition and focusing on the quality of fats and carbohydrates consumed, rather than strictly adhering to low-fat guidelines, Individuals can enhance their general health while lowering their risk of chronic disease.

Chapter 7

Beyond Calories: Hormones, Metabolism, and Weight Regulation

In today's dietary landscape, the focus on weight management often revolves around the simple equation of calories in versus calories out. While this concept is foundational, it oversimplifies the complex interplay between hormones, metabolism, and weight regulation. In this chapter, we delve deeper into the hormonal impact of processed foods on metabolism and weight regulation, explore the concept of insulin resistance and its role in metabolic syndrome, and emphasize the significance of food quality beyond calorie quantity for achieving optimal health.

The Hormonal Impact of Processed Foods

When we consume food, our bodies initiate a series of complex biochemical processes to metabolize and utilize nutrients. However, not all foods are created equal in terms of their hormonal effects. Processed foods, characterized by their high levels of refined sugars, unhealthy fats, and artificial additives, can significantly disrupt hormonal balance and metabolic function.

One of the primary hormones affected by processed foods is insulin. The pancreas produces insulin as a response to increased blood glucose levels following a meal. Its primary role is to facilitate the uptake of glucose into cells for energy production or storage. However, chronically elevated insulin levels, which commonly occur with the consumption of processed carbohydrates and sugars, can lead to insulin resistance.

Insulin resistance occurs when cells become less responsive to the effects of insulin, causing blood sugar levels to remain elevated. This metabolic dysfunction not only promotes fat storage but also contributes to a cascade of adverse health effects, including increased risk of type 2 diabetes, cardiovascular disease, and obesity.

Moreover, processed foods can disrupt the balance of other key hormones involved in appetite regulation and metabolism, such as leptin and ghrelin. Leptin, often referred to as the "satiety hormone," signals to the brain when we are full and should stop eating. Ghrelin, on the other hand, is known as the "hunger hormone" and stimulates appetite. Consuming processed foods high in refined sugars and unhealthy fats can dysregulate these hormones, leading to increased hunger, cravings, and overeating.

Furthermore, processed foods often lack essential nutrients and fiber, further exacerbating hormonal imbalances and metabolic dysfunction. For example, fiber plays a crucial role in regulating blood sugar levels and promoting satiety, yet it is typically deficient in processed foods.

Insulin Resistance and Metabolic Syndrome

Insulin resistance lies at the heart of metabolic syndrome, a cluster of conditions that significantly increase the risk of heart disease, stroke, and type 2 diabetes. Metabolic syndrome is diagnosed when an individual exhibits at least three of the following criteria: abdominal obesity, elevated blood pressure, high blood sugar, high triglycerides, and low HDL cholesterol levels.

The development of insulin resistance is closely linked to lifestyle factors, particularly diet and physical activity levels. Processed foods, which are high in refined carbohydrates and sugars, are major contributors to insulin resistance and metabolic syndrome. When consumed in excess, these foods trigger large spikes in blood sugar and insulin levels, placing undue stress on the body's insulin-regulating mechanisms.

Over time, the pancreas may struggle to maintain sufficient insulin production to overcome insulin resistance, leading to chronically elevated blood sugar levels. This condition, known as prediabetes, often precedes the onset of type 2 diabetes. Additionally, insulin resistance promotes the accumulation of visceral fat, particularly around the abdomen, which further exacerbates metabolic dysfunction and increases the risk of cardiovascular disease.

Moreover, insulin resistance is associated with systemic inflammation and oxidative stress, which play key roles in the pathogenesis of metabolic syndrome. Inflammatory processes disrupt normal metabolic signaling pathways, contributing to insulin resistance, impaired glucose tolerance, and dyslipidemia.

Fortunately, insulin resistance and metabolic syndrome are largely reversible through lifestyle modifications, particularly dietary changes and increased physical activity. By reducing the consumption of processed foods high in refined sugars and unhealthy fats, and instead focusing on whole, nutrient-dense foods, individuals can improve insulin sensitivity, regulate blood sugar levels, and mitigate the risk of metabolic syndrome and its associated complications.

The Importance of Food Quality

While calorie counting has long been the cornerstone of weight management strategies, emerging research suggests that the quality of calories consumed plays a critical role in metabolic health. Not all calories are metabolized equally, and the source of those calories can have profound effects on hormones, metabolism, and overall health outcomes.

Processed foods, despite their often low-calorie density, are notorious for their detrimental effects on metabolic health. These foods are typically high in refined sugars, unhealthy fats, and synthetic additives, which can disrupt hormonal balance, promote inflammation, and impair metabolic function.

In contrast, whole, nutrient-dense foods provide a wealth of essential nutrients, including vitamins, minerals, antioxidants, and dietary fiber, that are crucial for optimal health. These foods are minimally processed and retain their natural integrity, offering sustained energy, satiety, and metabolic support.

Furthermore, the quality of carbohydrates consumed plays a significant role in metabolic health. Refined carbohydrates, such as those found in white bread, sugary snacks, and sweetened beverages, are rapidly digested and absorbed, causing sharp spikes in blood sugar and insulin levels. In contrast, complex carbohydrates found in whole grains, fruits, vegetables, and legumes are digested more slowly, providing a steady source of energy and promoting stable blood sugar levels.

Similarly, the type of fats consumed can impact metabolic health. While processed foods often contain unhealthy trans fats and excessive amounts of omega-6 fatty acids, whole foods such as nuts, seeds, avocados, and fatty fish provide beneficial omega-3 fatty acids and monounsaturated fats that support cardiovascular health and metabolic function.

Prioritizing food quality over calorie quantity is essential for achieving and maintaining optimal health. By focusing on whole, nutrient-dense foods and minimizing the consumption of processed foods, individuals can support hormonal balance, regulate metabolism, and reduce the risk of chronic disease.

Chapter 8

The Industrialization of Agriculture

The Industrialization of Agriculture has transformed the way we produce food, shaping the landscape of modern farming practices and raising critical questions about sustainability, health, and environmental impact. This chapter explores the profound changes brought about by the Green Revolution, the widespread use of pesticides, herbicides, and GMOs, and the emerging sustainable alternatives for food production.

The Green Revolution and Its Consequences

The Green Revolution, a period of agricultural innovation that began in the mid-20th century, is hailed as a significant milestone in global food production. Its primary goals were to increase agricultural productivity and combat hunger by introducing high-yielding crop varieties, synthetic fertilizers, and pesticides.

At the heart of the Green Revolution were technological advancements that promised to boost crop yields and alleviate food shortages. High-yielding crop varieties, such as dwarf wheat and rice, were developed through selective breeding and genetic manipulation to produce more significant quantities of grains per acre.

The impact of the Green Revolution on global food production was monumental. Crop yields soared, leading to a substantial increase in food availability and a reduction in hunger in many parts of the world. Countries like India, Mexico, and the Philippines experienced remarkable agricultural growth, transforming from food-deficient nations to self-sufficient producers.

However, the Green Revolution was not without its consequences and criticisms. While it succeeded in increasing food production, it also led to significant environmental and social challenges.

One of the most pressing concerns is the reliance on chemical inputs such as synthetic fertilizers and pesticides. The widespread use of these chemicals has led to soil degradation, water pollution, and loss of biodiversity. Moreover, the intensive monoculture farming practices promoted by the Green Revolution have contributed to the erosion of genetic diversity, making crops more vulnerable to pests, diseases, and climate change.

Another criticism of the Green Revolution is its uneven distribution of benefits. While some regions and farmers have reaped the rewards of increased productivity, others have been left behind, exacerbating inequalities within the agricultural sector. Small-scale farmers, in particular, have struggled to compete in a system dominated by large agribusinesses and multinational corporations.

Despite its shortcomings, the Green Revolution has undoubtedly shaped the trajectory of global agriculture. Its legacy continues to influence agricultural policies, research priorities, and investment decisions around the world. As we grapple with the challenges of feeding a growing population in a sustainable manner, it is essential to critically evaluate the lessons learned from the Green Revolution and explore alternative pathways for food production.

Pesticides, Herbicides, and GMOs

The widespread use of pesticides, herbicides, and genetically modified organisms (GMOs) has become synonymous with modern agriculture, promising increased yields, pest resistance, and weed control. However, the indiscriminate use of these chemical inputs has raised significant concerns about their impact on human health, the environment, and biodiversity.

Pesticides, including insecticides, herbicides, and fungicides, are chemicals used to control pests and diseases in crops. While they have been instrumental in protecting crops from damage and increasing yields, their overuse has led to adverse effects on non-target organisms, including beneficial insects, birds, and aquatic life.

Moreover, there is growing evidence linking pesticide exposure to a range of human health problems, including cancer, neurological disorders, and reproductive issues. Vulnerable populations, such as farmworkers and rural communities, are disproportionately affected by pesticide exposure, highlighting the social injustices inherent in industrial agriculture.

Herbicides, specifically designed to control weeds, have also come under scrutiny for their environmental and health impacts. Glyphosate, the active ingredient in the popular herbicide Roundup, has been classified as a probable human carcinogen by the International Agency for Research on Cancer (IARC). Its widespread use has led to the emergence of glyphosate-resistant weeds, exacerbating the problem of weed control and driving farmers to use even more potent herbicides.

Genetically modified organisms (GMOs) represent another controversial aspect of modern agriculture. Engineered to possess specific traits such as herbicide tolerance or pest resistance, GMOs have been heralded as a solution to global food security challenges. However, concerns about the long-term environmental and health effects of GMOs persist, with critics warning of unintended consequences such as gene flow to wild relatives and the development of resistance in target pests.

Despite these concerns, the adoption of GMOs continues to grow, driven by the interests of agribusiness giants and policymakers who view biotechnology as a tool for increasing agricultural productivity and profitability. However, as we confront the challenges of climate change, soil degradation, and biodiversity loss, it is imperative to reassess our reliance on chemical-intensive farming practices and explore alternative approaches to sustainable agriculture.

Sustainable Alternatives for Food Production

In recent years, there has been a growing recognition of the need to transition towards more sustainable and regenerative farming practices that prioritize environmental stewardship, soil health, and biodiversity conservation. A variety of alternative approaches to food production have emerged, offering promising solutions to the challenges posed by industrial agriculture.

Agroecology, often described as the science of sustainable agriculture, emphasizes the integration of ecological principles into farming systems. By harnessing natural processes such as nutrient cycling, biological pest control, and soil fertility management, agroecological practices seek to enhance resilience, productivity, and biodiversity while reducing reliance on external inputs.

Organic farming represents another sustainable alternative to conventional agriculture, focusing on the use of natural inputs and holistic management practices to promote soil health and ecosystem balance. Organic farmers eschew synthetic pesticides, herbicides, and fertilizers in favor of organic alternatives such as compost, cover crops, and crop rotation.

Permaculture, a design philosophy inspired by natural ecosystems, seeks to create self-sustaining agricultural systems that mimic the resilience and diversity of natural ecosystems. By incorporating principles such as diversity, observation, and integration, permaculture practitioners aim to design productive landscapes that are both ecologically sound and economically viable.

In addition to these alternative farming systems, there is growing interest in agroforestry, regenerative agriculture, and community-supported agriculture (CSA) as means of promoting sustainable food production and resilient food systems. These approaches prioritize collaboration, knowledge sharing, and community engagement, fostering connections between farmers, consumers, and the land.

As we confront the challenges of feeding a growing population in a changing climate, it is clear that the future of food production lies in sustainable, regenerative, and equitable agricultural systems. By embracing diverse approaches to farming and investing in agroecological research, education, and policy support, we can build a food system that nourishes both people and the planet for generations to come.

Chapter 9

The Medicalization of Food

In today's world, the intersection of food, nutrition, and medicine has become increasingly complex. One of the most significant phenomena shaping this intersection is the medicalization of food. This chapter delves deep into the influence of pharmaceutical companies on nutrition research and dietary guidelines, critiques the use of medications as a band-aid solution for dietary diseases, and explores integrative approaches to health and healing that prioritize nutrition and lifestyle interventions.

The Influence of Pharmaceutical Companies on Nutrition Research

The relationship between pharmaceutical companies and nutrition research is intricate and often contentious. While the primary aim of pharmaceutical companies is to develop and market drugs for various health conditions, their influence extends into other domains, including nutrition research.

Pharmaceutical Funding of Research

Pharmaceutical companies frequently fund research studies related to nutrition and health. While this funding can accelerate scientific discovery and innovation, it also raises concerns about conflicts of interest and bias. Studies funded by pharmaceutical companies may be more likely to produce results favorable to their products or interests, potentially skewing the evidence base.

Moreover, pharmaceutical funding may prioritize research on drug interventions over non-pharmacological approaches such as diet and lifestyle modifications. This bias can shape the research agenda, leading to an imbalance in the evidence available to guide clinical practice and public health policies.

Influence on Dietary Guidelines

The influence of pharmaceutical companies extends to the development of dietary guidelines, which play a crucial role in shaping public health recommendations and policies. Pharmaceutical interests may exert indirect influence through professional associations, advocacy groups, and industry-funded research that informs the formulation of dietary guidelines.

Conflicts of interest among expert panel members tasked with developing dietary guidelines have also come under scrutiny. Many panel members have financial ties to pharmaceutical companies or food industry organizations, raising questions about the impartiality and independence of guideline recommendations.

Furthermore, pharmaceutical companies may engage in lobbying and advocacy efforts to promote policies favorable to their products, such as the inclusion of pharmaceutical interventions in dietary guidelines or the regulation of dietary supplements that compete with pharmaceutical drugs.

Critique of Medications as a Band-Aid Solution for Dietary Diseases

In the treatment of dietary diseases such as obesity, type 2 diabetes, and cardiovascular disorders, medications are often used as a primary or adjunct therapy. While medications can effectively manage symptoms and complications associated with these conditions, they often serve as a band-aid solution rather than addressing the underlying dietary and lifestyle factors driving disease development.

Symptom Management vs. Root Cause Resolution

Medications used to treat dietary diseases typically target specific physiological pathways or symptoms associated with the condition. For example, antihypertensive drugs may lower blood pressure, while antidiabetic medications help regulate blood glucose levels. While these interventions can provide symptomatic relief and improve quality of life, they do not address the root causes of the diseases.

Side Effects and Long-Term Risks

Like all medications, drugs used to treat dietary diseases carry potential side effects and long-term risks. Common side effects may include gastrointestinal disturbances, dizziness, fatigue, and weight gain, among others. In some cases, the long-term use of medications may be associated with more serious adverse effects, including organ damage, metabolic disturbances, and increased risk of other health conditions.

Moreover, relying solely on medications to manage dietary diseases may foster a sense of complacency and dependency, detracting from efforts to implement lifestyle modifications and behavioral changes that address the root causes of the conditions.

Economic and Societal Implications
The widespread use of medications to treat dietary diseases has significant economic and societal implications. Healthcare expenditures related to pharmaceutical interventions for dietary diseases are substantial, placing a burden on healthcare systems and taxpayers.

Additionally, the medicalization of food contributes to a culture of pill-popping and quick-fix solutions, perpetuating the misconception that health can be achieved solely through medical interventions rather than holistic lifestyle approaches.

Integrative Approaches to Health and Healing

In contrast to the medicalization of food, integrative approaches to health and healing emphasize a comprehensive, patient-centered approach that addresses the interconnectedness of mind, body, and spirit. These approaches prioritize nutrition and lifestyle interventions as foundational components of health promotion and disease prevention.

Holistic Health Paradigm

Integrative medicine embraces a holistic health paradigm that recognizes the importance of addressing the underlying causes of disease rather than merely suppressing symptoms. This paradigm emphasizes the body's innate healing capacity and seeks to support and optimize its natural processes through personalized interventions tailored to each individual's unique needs and circumstances.

Nutritional Medicine

Nutritional medicine is a cornerstone of integrative approaches to health, emphasizing the therapeutic potential of food as medicine. Dietary interventions, including personalized nutrition plans, dietary supplements, and functional foods, are used to promote optimal health, prevent disease, and support the treatment of various health conditions.

Lifestyle Medicine

Lifestyle medicine focuses on modifying lifestyle factors such as diet, physical activity, stress management, sleep, and social support to prevent and treat chronic diseases. Lifestyle interventions are evidence-based, and cost-effective, and empower individuals to take an active role in their health and well-being.

Mind-Body Therapies

Mind-body therapies, including meditation, yoga, tai chi, and mindfulness-based stress reduction, promote relaxation, reduce stress, and enhance emotional well-being. These practices have been shown to positively impact physiological processes, immune function, and overall health outcomes.

Integrative Healthcare Models

Integrative healthcare models, such as functional medicine and naturopathic medicine, combine conventional medical approaches with complementary and alternative therapies to provide comprehensive, patient-centered care. These models emphasize the importance of treating the whole person rather than focusing solely on symptoms or disease labels.

The medicalization of food represents a paradigm shift in how we approach health and healing, with profound implications for individuals, communities, and societies. By critically examining the influence of pharmaceutical companies on nutrition research and dietary guidelines, questioning the use of medications as a band-aid solution for dietary diseases, and exploring integrative approaches to health and healing, we can foster a more holistic and sustainable approach to health that prioritizes nutrition, lifestyle interventions, and personalized care.

Chapter 10

Navigating the Food Landscape:

Practical Solutions for a Healthier Future

In this chapter, we delve into actionable strategies for individuals and communities to navigate the complex food landscape and cultivate healthier eating habits. By addressing the challenges posed by processed foods, advocating for the consumption of whole foods, and promoting policy changes and food system reform, we can collectively work towards a healthier future.

Strategies for Reducing Processed Food Consumption

Processed foods have become pervasive in our modern food environment, often tempting us with their convenience and palatability. However, their consumption is associated with a myriad of health issues, including obesity, diabetes, and heart disease. To combat the detrimental effects of processed foods, it's essential to adopt strategies that prioritize whole, minimally processed foods.

1. Meal Planning and Preparation:

One of the most effective ways to reduce reliance on processed foods is by planning and preparing meals at home. Set aside time each week to plan your meals, make a grocery list, and prep ingredients in advance. By having nutritious meals readily available, you'll be less likely to reach for processed options when hunger strikes.

2. Focus on Whole Ingredients: When grocery shopping, prioritize whole foods such as fruits, vegetables, whole grains, legumes, and lean proteins. These nutrient-dense foods not only nourish your body but also help reduce cravings for processed snacks and junk foods.

3. Read Food Labels: Take the time to read food labels and familiarize yourself with common additives, preservatives, and artificial ingredients found in processed foods. Opt for products with short ingredient lists and avoid those containing high levels of added sugars, unhealthy fats, and artificial additives.

4. Cook from Scratch: Embrace the art of cooking from scratch using whole ingredients. Experiment with different recipes and cooking techniques to create delicious and satisfying meals that are free from processed ingredients. Get creative in the kitchen and involve your family members or friends to make cooking a fun and enjoyable experience.

5. Limit Convenience Foods: While convenient, pre-packaged and ready-to-eat foods are often loaded with unhealthy additives and preservatives. Minimize your consumption of convenience foods such as frozen meals, snack bars, and fast food by opting for homemade alternatives whenever possible.

6. Practice Mindful Eating: Slow down and pay attention to your body's hunger and fullness cues when eating. Mindful eating can help prevent overeating and reduce the urge to snack on processed foods out of boredom or stress.

7. Stock a Healthy Pantry: Keep your pantry stocked with nutritious staples such as whole grains, canned beans, nuts, seeds, and healthy cooking oils. Having a well-stocked pantry makes it easier to whip up healthy meals and snacks without relying on processed foods.

8. Choose Whole-Food Snacks: When hunger strikes between meals, reach for whole-food snacks such as fresh fruit, raw vegetables with hummus, nuts, or yogurt instead of processed snacks like chips, cookies, or candy.

9. Stay Hydrated: Sometimes, thirst can masquerade as hunger, leading to unnecessary snacking on processed foods. Stay hydrated by drinking plenty of water throughout the day and opt for water or herbal tea instead of sugary beverages.

10. Practice Moderation: While it's important to prioritize whole foods, it's also okay to enjoy processed treats occasionally in moderation. Allow yourself the flexibility to indulge in your favorite processed foods on occasion without guilt, but make whole, nutritious foods the foundation of your diet.

By implementing these strategies, you can gradually reduce your reliance on processed foods and transition towards a diet that prioritizes whole, nutrient-dense ingredients, leading to improved health and well-being.

The Value of Whole Foods and Home Cooking

Whole foods are the cornerstone of a healthy diet, providing essential nutrients that nourish our bodies and support optimal health. In contrast to processed foods, which are often stripped of their natural nutrients and loaded with unhealthy additives, whole foods are minimally processed or refined, retaining their nutritional integrity. Home cooking allows us to harness the nutritional power of whole foods while fostering a deeper connection to the food we eat.

1. Nutrient Density: Whole foods are high in critical nutrients such vitamins, minerals, fiber, and antioxidants, all of which are important for overall health and preventing chronic diseases. By incorporating a variety of whole foods into your diet, you can ensure that your body receives the nutrients it needs to thrive.

2. Disease Prevention: Numerous studies have demonstrated the health benefits of consuming a diet rich in whole foods. Diets high in fruits, vegetables, whole grains, and lean proteins have been associated with a lower risk of obesity, heart disease, diabetes, and certain types of cancer. By prioritizing whole foods, you can reduce your risk of developing chronic diseases and promote longevity.

3. Improved Digestion: Whole foods are typically higher in fiber than processed foods, which can promote healthy digestion and regular bowel movements. Fiber helps to bulk up stools, regulate bowel movements, and support the growth of beneficial gut bacteria. By incorporating fiber-rich whole foods such as fruits, vegetables, whole grains, and legumes into your diet, you can support optimal digestive health.

4. Weight Management: Whole foods are often lower in calories and higher in nutrients than processed foods, making them a valuable tool for weight management. By focusing on whole, minimally processed foods, you can feel satisfied and satiated while consuming fewer calories, making it easier to maintain a healthy weight.

5. Environmental Sustainability: Choosing whole foods that are locally sourced and sustainably produced can have positive impacts on the environment. By supporting small-scale farmers and sustainable agricultural practices, you can help reduce the carbon footprint of your diet and promote environmental sustainability.

6. Cultural Connection: Home cooking allows us to celebrate our cultural heritage and connect with our families and communities through food. Sharing meals prepared with love and care fosters a sense of belonging and strengthens bonds with loved ones.

7. Budget-Friendly: Contrary to popular belief, cooking meals at home with whole ingredients can be more cost-effective than relying on processed foods or dining out. By purchasing seasonal produce, buying in bulk, and planning meals in advance, you can save money while nourishing your body with wholesome, nutritious foods.

8. Enhanced Flavor and Satisfaction: Whole foods are bursting with natural flavors and textures that can elevate the taste and enjoyment of your meals.

Experimenting with fresh herbs, spices, and cooking techniques can enhance the flavor of whole foods and make home-cooked meals more satisfying and delicious.

9. Empowerment and Independence: Learning to cook simple, nourishing meals at home empowers individuals to take control of their health and well-being. By developing culinary skills and confidence in the kitchen, you can become more self-sufficient and independent when it comes to feeding yourself and your family.

10. Mindful Eating: Home cooking encourages mindfulness and presence during mealtime, allowing you to savor and appreciate the flavors, textures, and aromas of your food. By slowing down and enjoying your meals without distractions, you can cultivate a deeper connection to the food you eat and enhance your overall eating experience.

By prioritizing whole, minimally processed ingredients and embracing the art of cooking at home, you can nourish your body, support your health goals, and cultivate a deeper appreciation for food and its role in your life.

Advocacy for Policy Change and Food System Reform

The food we eat is not only a personal choice but also a reflection of larger societal and environmental factors. Our current food system is rife with issues ranging from food insecurity and inequity to environmental degradation and public health crises. Advocating for policy change and food system reform is essential to address these systemic challenges and create a more just, sustainable, and equitable food system for all.

1. Addressing Food Insecurity:

Millions of people around the world lack access

to nutritious, affordable food, leading to food insecurity and malnutrition. By advocating for policies that prioritize food access, affordability, and equity, we can work towards ensuring that everyone has access to the nutritious food they need to thrive.

2. Supporting Local Farmers and Producers: Small-scale farmers and producers play a vital role in our food system, yet they often face numerous challenges, including limited access to markets and resources. By advocating for policies that support local agriculture, such as farm-to-school programs, farmers' markets, and land preservation initiatives, we can strengthen local food systems and support the livelihoods of farmers and producers in our communities.

3. Promoting Sustainable Agriculture: Conventional agriculture practices have negative impacts on soil health, water quality, and biodiversity, contributing to

environmental degradation and climate change. By advocating for policies that promote sustainable agriculture practices, such as organic farming, regenerative agriculture, and agroecology, we can mitigate these impacts and build a more resilient and sustainable food system.

4. Regulating Food Marketing and Advertising

The food industry often uses marketing and advertising tactics to promote unhealthy foods and beverages, particularly to children and adolescents. By advocating for policies that regulate food marketing and advertising, such as restrictions on junk food advertising targeted at children and the implementation of front-of-package labeling systems, we can protect public health and empower consumers to make informed choices about the foods they eat.

5. Improving School Food Programs

School food programs play a

critical role in shaping children's eating habits and overall health. By advocating for policies that improve the quality and nutritional content of school meals, increase access to fresh, locally sourced foods, and provide nutrition education and cooking skills training, we can support the health and well-being of our nation's youth.

6. Addressing Food Waste: Food waste is a significant issue that contributes to environmental degradation, economic losses, and food insecurity. By advocating for policies that promote food waste reduction and diversion efforts, such as standardized date labeling, food recovery programs, and composting initiatives, we can reduce waste throughout the food supply chain and create a more sustainable and efficient food system.

7. Fostering Food Sovereignty: Food sovereignty is the right of people to control their own food systems, including the production, distribution, and consumption of food. By advocating for policies that prioritize food sovereignty, such as land reform, seed sovereignty, and community-based food systems, we can empower communities to reclaim control over their food systems and build resilience against external threats.

8. Supporting Food Justice: Food justice is the equitable distribution of healthy, culturally appropriate food to all people, regardless of race, ethnicity, income, or geography. By advocating for policies that address systemic inequalities and barriers to food access, such as anti-hunger initiatives, fair labor practices, and racial equity in food systems, we can work towards creating a more just and inclusive food system for all.

9. Engaging in Advocacy and Activism: As individuals and communities, we have the power to advocate for positive change in our food system through grassroots activism, community organizing, and political

engagement. By raising awareness, mobilizing support, and holding policymakers and food industry stakeholders accountable, we can create momentum for meaningful policy change and food system reform.

10. Building Coalitions and Partnerships: Collaboration and partnership are essential for driving collective action and creating lasting change in our food system. By building coalitions with diverse stakeholders, including farmers, producers, consumers, advocacy groups, and policymakers, we can leverage our collective expertise, resources, and influence to advance shared goals and priorities.

Advocating for policy change and food system reform is critical to addressing the systemic challenges facing our current food system and creating a more sustainable, equitable, and resilient food system for future generations. By working together and advocating for policies that prioritize food access, sustainability, and

justice, we can create positive change and build
a healthier, more vibrant food system for all.

Conclusion

Throughout the pages of "Metabolical Maelstrom: Exposing the Deception in Processed Foods, Nutrition, and Medical Practices" we embarked on a journey of discovery, unraveling the intricate web that connects our food choices, nutrition, and health outcomes. We delved deep into the seductive allure of processed foods, dissected the nutritional myths perpetuated by the modern food industry, and explored the profound impact of our dietary habits on our bodies and minds. As we draw near the end of this enlightening exploration, it's crucial to reflect on the key insights and arguments that have unfolded before us.

Summarizing Key Insights and Arguments

In our investigation, we unearthed the stark realities of the Western diet a diet characterized by the overconsumption of processed foods laden with sugars, unhealthy fats, and synthetic additives. We witnessed how this diet has fueled an epidemic of obesity, diabetes, cardiovascular disease, and other chronic health conditions, exacting a heavy toll on individuals and societies alike. Through compelling evidence and real-life stories, we exposed the deceptive marketing tactics employed by the processed food industry to perpetuate a cycle of addiction and dependency, all while prioritizing profits over public health.

Moreover, we challenged prevailing nutritional dogmas, debunking the myth that all calories are created equal and shedding light on the crucial role of nutrient density in promoting optimal health. We explored the intricate interplay between the gut microbiome and overall well-being, underscoring the importance of nurturing our inner ecosystem through wholesome, unprocessed foods. Additionally, we examined the detrimental effects of sugar consumption on metabolic health and delved into the truth about dietary fats, dispelling misconceptions surrounding their role in heart disease.

Furthermore, we ventured into the realm of agricultural industrialization, uncovering the hidden costs of modern farming practices on both human health and the environment. From the pervasive use of pesticides and herbicides to the proliferation of genetically modified organisms (GMOs), we confronted the stark reality of a food system in crisis. Yet, amidst these challenges, we also discovered glimmers of hope sustainable alternatives, and regenerative farming practices that offer a path forward toward a healthier, more resilient food system.

The Importance of Viewing Food as Medicine

Central to our journey is the recognition that food is not just fuel for our bodies but also a powerful form of medicine. Each bite we take has the potential to either nourish or harm us, promote health, or contribute to disease. By embracing this fundamental truth and adopting a holistic approach to health one that encompasses not only what we eat but also how we live we reclaim agency over our well-being.

Indeed, the concept of food as medicine extends beyond the realm of individual health to encompass broader societal implications. By prioritizing whole, unprocessed foods and supporting regenerative agriculture, we not only safeguard our own health but also contribute to the well-being of future generations and the planet as a whole. It is a profound act of self-care and planetary stewardship a declaration of our commitment to a more vibrant, sustainable future.

As we stand at the crossroads of possibility, poised to shape the future of our health and our planet, it is incumbent upon each of us to take action. We must become catalysts for change in our own lives and communities, advocating for policies and practices that prioritize health, equity, and sustainability. Whether it's choosing to support local farmers and artisans, advocating for better food access in underserved communities, or participating in grassroots movements for food system reform, every action we take matters.

Moreover, we must recognize the power of our collective voices to effect change on a larger scale. By joining forces with like-minded individuals and organizations, we amplify our impact and create a ripple effect of positive change that reverberates far and wide. Together, we have the power to reshape our food system, reclaim our health, and create a world where nutritious, wholesome food is not just a privilege but a fundamental human right.

In closing, "Metabolical" serves as both a wake-up call and a call to action a rallying cry for all those who believe in the transformative power of food to heal, nourish, and sustain us. Let us heed this call with courage, conviction, and compassion, knowing that the choices we make today have the power to shape the health and well-being of generations to come. Together, let us reclaim our health and chart a course toward a brighter, healthier future for all.